Jagdeep Virk
Bhik Kotecha

Radiofrequency thermal ablation for sleep-related disordered breathing

AF153152

Jagdeep Virk
Bhik Kotecha

Radiofrequency thermal ablation for sleep-related disordered breathing

LAP LAMBERT Academic Publishing

Impressum / Imprint

Bibliografische Information der Deutschen Nationalbibliothek: Die Deutsche Nationalbibliothek verzeichnet diese Publikation in der Deutschen Nationalbibliografie; detaillierte bibliografische Daten sind im Internet über http://dnb.d-nb.de abrufbar.

Alle in diesem Buch genannten Marken und Produktnamen unterliegen warenzeichen-, marken- oder patentrechtlichem Schutz bzw. sind Warenzeichen oder eingetragene Warenzeichen der jeweiligen Inhaber. Die Wiedergabe von Marken, Produktnamen, Gebrauchsnamen, Handelsnamen, Warenbezeichnungen u.s.w. in diesem Werk berechtigt auch ohne besondere Kennzeichnung nicht zu der Annahme, dass solche Namen im Sinne der Warenzeichen- und Markenschutzgesetzgebung als frei zu betrachten wären und daher von jedermann benutzt werden dürften.

Bibliographic information published by the Deutsche Nationalbibliothek: The Deutsche Nationalbibliothek lists this publication in the Deutsche Nationalbibliografie; detailed bibliographic data are available in the Internet at http://dnb.d-nb.de.

Any brand names and product names mentioned in this book are subject to trademark, brand or patent protection and are trademarks or registered trademarks of their respective holders. The use of brand names, product names, common names, trade names, product descriptions etc. even without a particular marking in this work is in no way to be construed to mean that such names may be regarded as unrestricted in respect of trademark and brand protection legislation and could thus be used by anyone.

Coverbild / Cover image: www.ingimage.com

Verlag / Publisher:
LAP LAMBERT Academic Publishing
ist ein Imprint der / is a trademark of
OmniScriptum GmbH & Co. KG
Heinrich-Böcking-Str. 6-8, 66121 Saarbrücken, Deutschland / Germany
Email: info@lap-publishing.com

Herstellung: siehe letzte Seite /
Printed at: see last page
ISBN: 978-3-659-79053-9

The role of radiofrequency thermal ablation in sleep-related disordered breathing

Jagdeep S Virk[*] MA MRCS DOHNS and Bhik Kotecha[*] MPhil FRCS DLO

[*]Royal National Throat Nose & Ear Hospital, London

Address for correspondence: *Bhik Kotecha, Consultant Otolaryngologist, Royal National Throat, Nose & Ear Hospital, 330 Grays Inn Road, London WC1X 8DA,* bhikkot@aol.com

Index

Abstract

Sleep-related disordered breathing is increasingly prevalent. Management of these patients is complex and requires a multidisciplinary team including respiratory physicians, otolaryngologists and maxillo-facial surgeons. Treatment strategies are often used in combination and target multilevel obstruction sites. As such, management is individually tailored and careful patient selection is necessary.

Radiofrequency thermal ablation has been one of the most promising surgical options for patients in the last decade. We perform a thorough review of its concept, basis, surgical technique and long term efficacy.

Key words: snoring, obstructive sleep apnoea, radiofrequency ablation

Introduction

Sleep-related disordered breathing (SRDB) refers to a spectrum of diagnoses, ranging from simple snoring to severe obstructive sleep apnoea. Within the continuum lie other disorders such as obesity-induced hypoventilation and upper airway resistance syndrome. The shared underlying diagnostic feature is that of recurrent partial or complete cessation of breathing.[1] The most common of these conditions remain snoring and obstructive sleep apnoea.

Epidemiological studies and self-reported surveys indicate that the prevalence of snoring is in the range of 25-50 % for middle aged men (in a 2:1 ratio with women), while obstructive sleep apnoea (OSA) affects 2-4 % of males and 1-2 % of females, a rate comparable with Type 1 Diabetes.[2-6] However a large proportion of cases are undiagnosed, with one study in a US community of almost 5000 patients demonstrating that up to 82 % of males and 92 % of females likely to have moderate or severe OSA had not yet been diagnosed.[7] With the ensuing obesity epidemic, SRDB will only increase in prevalence and serve as a significant health and socio-economic burden.[8-10]

The pathophysiology of SRDB is complex and multifactorial, with a single cause rarely identified. Associations include obesity, increased neck circumference, craniofacial abnormalities and anatomical variations (e.g. retrognathia, macroglossia, nasal polyposis), hypothyroidism, acromegaly, family history, alcohol or sedative intake and body position.[11,12]

Sleep-related disordered breathing demonstrates an associated morbidity and mortality, particularly within the OSA subgroup, and this, in turn, correlates with a huge social and economic outlay. These conditions have been recognised as independent risk factors for cardiac arrhythmias, pulmonary and systemic hypertension, myocardial infarction, type 2 diabetes mellitus, cerebrovascular accidents, impaired cognition and road traffic accidents.[13-17] In addition, there is evidence that moderate-to-severe OSA is independently associated with a large increased risk of all-cause mortality.[12,18] As a corollary to this, a recent study confirmed that untreated OSA increases healthcare utilisation, occupational injuries and reduces work performance, resulting in a substantial socio-economic impact in the order of billions of dollars per year.[8]

Management of this subset of patients is complex and involves a multidisciplinary team. Patient selection is the critical factor and this is dependent upon a thorough clinical evaluation and work up.[19] Over the last two decades, there has been increasing interest and advancements in the surgical treatment of patients with snoring and OSA, particularly in the role of radiofrequency thermal ablation.[20-23] Longer term studies alongside meta-analyses are demonstrating the efficacy of this technique and this review article summarises the current literature and up to date clinical tips and pitfalls of the surgical technique alongside its scientific basis.

Basic science

Radio frequency specifically refers to a range of electromagnetic wave frequencies from 3 kHz to 300 GHz. In accordance with Faraday's law of electromagnetic induction, these radio waves or electric current can be utilised to generate thermal energy. For medical purposes, the typical ranges for radiofrequency thermal ablation are from 350 to 500 kHz. Radiofrequency technology entails the patient being part of a circuit, with a radiofrequency generator and a disposable hand piece. The thermal energy generated (55-90 ^{0}C) by the high frequency alternating current can be used to cut *and* coagulate.

Radiofrequency ablation (RFA) is minimally invasive and can be applied interstitially or in cutting mode. Snoring surgery is typically multilevel to the upper airway and as such, the radiofrequency application is well suited to this methodology, allowing concomitant applications for both resection of redundant palatopharyngeus mucosa and coagulation to the inferior turbinate, soft palate and base of tongue.[19,24] RFA is available in both monopolar and bipolar formats, although bipolar is preferable as it is associated with less energy deliverance and precise placement of the radiofrequency probes. Moreover, these devices can be impedance or temperature-modulated. RF works by causing ionic agitation of the tissues surrounding the probe, which in turn results in frictional heat and thermal energy.[25]

The main advantage of radiofrequency current is its inherent safety profile, as compared to previously used low frequency alternating current or pulsed direct current. Radiofrequency current does not directly stimulate nerves or muscle, thereby allowing application under local anaesthetic, although in many centres patient preference remains general anaesthetic. In addition, it is thought that RFA generates very little collateral tissue damage and hence reduced side effects and pain. This will be discussed in depth later.

Histopathological effects

A detailed understanding of the histological and ultrastructural effects of cutting and coagulative RFA allows appropriate surgical planning. As with all surgery, the outcome is operator dependent and so, an appreciation of these cellular effects during surgery, particularly lateral thermal spread and comparative studies with laser are imperative. There is however a paucity of literature in this field.

For cutting radiofrequency applications, Stimpson et al investigated the maximal depth of tissue injury and tissue type at this depth for patients undergoing uvula and posterior faucal pillar resection. This is the only study of human subjects to date. Of all the specimens, 19 of 30 (63 %) had a maximal injury depth of 0.1 mm or less. The overall mean maximal depth of injury was 0.15 mm. All specimens demonstrated fibrinoid changes at the resection margin with presence of dense eosinophilic material secondary to protein degeneration. The tissue type at the maximal depth was variable but was typically lamina propria. Ultrastructural analysis with electron microscopy indicated that RFA produced a more accurate cut when compared with carbon dioxide laser, with less shedding of squamous cells and preservation of submucosal tissue structures.[24] In conclusion, RFA electrosection caused little collateral soft tissue damage and appeared to be more accurate, with less concomitant trauma in comparison to carbon dioxide laser. This is in keeping with current thinking that radiofrequency procedures are minimally invasive, with reduced side effect profiles.

The principal study of histopathological effects of interstitial or coagulation RFA was undertaken by Virk et al on both human and animal tissue. Interstitial applications of

RFA generated a constant size of oval lesion in human tonsil tissue that was independent of power setting and local anaesthetic infiltration. This finding was reproduced in animal tissue, with a mean and median size of lesion of 7.9 x 6.4 mm (95 % CI: 7.7-8.1; 6.2-6.7) and 8 x 7 mm, respectively. Histopathological analysis confirmed submucosal lesions of significantly smaller magnitude (3 x 2 mm) but, significantly, no collateral damage beyond a distinct cut-off point, thereby ruling out diffuse tissue damage. Furthermore, it was noted that lower power settings generated denser lesions and more tissue reaction, but not beyond the cut-off transition point (Figure 1). In most radiofrequency devices, the power setting is inversely proportional to the energy delivered.[26]

Figure 1: representative slide of tonsil tissue demonstrating histological changes following application of 6 W (*left panel*) and 10 W (*right panel*) radiofrequency probe (H&E stain, x40 magnification). Note the lack of collateral damage beyond distinct cut off points (*black arrows*) and denser lesion in 6 W application.

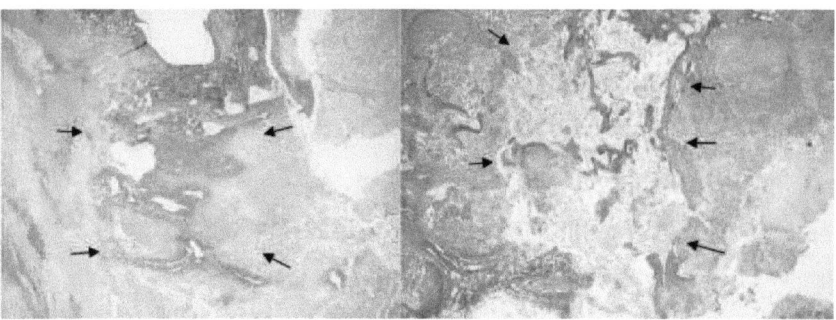

With kind permission from Springer Science and Business Media: [26]*Virk JS, Kumar G, Al-Okati D, Kotecha B. Radiofrequency ablation in snoring surgery: local tissue effects and safety measures. Eur Arch Otorhinolaryngol 2014; 271:3313-3318.*

Radiofrequency usage is continuously increasing in medicine. With all new techniques, a greater understanding of its mode of action alongside adequate training will improve its application, reliability, outcomes and reduce complications.[26] As a result of this study, introduction of local anaesthetic is recommended into the soft palate prior to RFA as it increases interstitial volume, improves ease of access but still does not affect the size of the lesion, hence serving as a safety measure (alongside providing some haemostasis). In addition, due to the width of the demonstrated RFA lesions along with further experiments in animal tissue, the authors demonstrated that contiguous lesions should be at least 8 mm apart to avoid submucosal/deeper tissue damage by coalescence of lesions, hence reducing the risk of ulceration and fistulation. This study also highlights that the number of radiofrequency applications can vary and is determined by the length and breadth of the soft palate and exposure of the region posterior to the circumvallate papillae at the tongue base.[26]

RF works by causing ionic agitation of the tissues surrounding the probe, which in turn results in frictional heat and thermal energy.[25] Desinger et al demonstrated that the volume and shape of coagulation necrosis induced depends upon the energy delivered, probe geometry, duration of thermal exposure, fluid content of the target tissue and blood vessel density.[27] In vivo, the heat-sink effect has to be considered.[28] The same team also demonstrated, in both animal and in vitro experiments, that carbonisation and dehydration can be avoided by irrigation of tissue during treatment and less power was required with the bipolar set up.[29]

Further work is required in this field as most studies are in animal tissue, in vitro, or have limitations such as the myriad radiofrequency devices and probes available, the time-dependent nature of fibrosis and hence histopathological change, and the varying types of tissue (e.g. palate, tongue base).

Radiological effects

The goals of surgery for the upper airway in patients with SRDB are to bypass upper airway obstruction, to increase the upper airway anatomical dimensions or to induce scarring/stiffening of the tissues. In addition, surgery may be performed to facilitate non-invasive ventilation (usually continuous positive airway pressure, CPAP), the gold standard treatment for OSA.

In light of this, serial imaging studies have sought to highlight the time-dependent nature of the tissue reaction alongside the extent to which RFA affects the upper airway dimensions. All studies employed the use of magnetic resonance imaging (MRI) and demonstrated that the RFA-induced lesions were visible immediately postoperatively. These studies elucidated areas of central hyperintensity, reflecting haemorrhagic, coagulative necrosis, surrounded by hypointensity, representing oedema, on T1-weighted images. The lesions initially expanded up to day three and then gradually diminished but were still evident at week six postoperatively.[30-32] Two of the studies focused on very early changes within 72 hours but confirmed the initial oedema and necrosis, in keeping with the histopathological findings described above, typical of wound healing following injury.[30,32] Heywood et al did however point towards a long term general trend towards an increase in airway dimensions. In a porcine study, Powell et al implied this time-dependent effect of reduction in tissue volume.[33] In a cephalometric study, with plain radiographs only, there is also evidence that airway dimensions are improved.[20]

Historical perspective

D'Arsonval, in 1891, was the first to have reported the heating effect of radiofrequency waves, and this, many years later, led to the evolution of devices such as electrocautery and ultimately, radiofrequency ablation.[34] This discovery lay relatively latent until the introduction of the Bovie knife in 1928 by Cushing and Bovie, which allowed cutting and cauterisation of tissue by varying the RF current.[35]

Since the 1970s, radiofrequency ablation has increasingly been employed in a wide variety of fields but initially found utility in cardiology to ablate arrhythmias. RFA procedures are typically performed under image guidance in these instances. A wide variety of applications have since developed including the treatment of tumours (initially the liver), parkinsonian tremors, trigeminal neuralgia, varicose veins and chronic pain.

In 1998, Powell et al first reported the role of radiofrequency ablation for SRDB patients in a pilot study of 22 patients.[20] Since then, publications and interest have proliferated such that RFA has an accepted role as a minimally invasive treatment for the multilevel obstructions typical of SRDB, including the inferior turbinates, soft palate and tongue base. The current research goals are to better define surgical outcomes, standardise nomenclature and build a clear evidence base for long term success.

Clinical evaluation

A critical factor in performing RFA surgery is patient selection, in that an accurate assessment and evaluation of the dynamics of the upper airway is required preoperatively to subsequently produce optimal patient outcomes.[19,26] However, this is often poorly conducted.

A thorough history, clinical examination and appropriate investigations are required prior to consideration of any intervention. The clinical history can be attained from both the patient and the partner or co-habitant, if relevant. This should include a description of the snoring and if any apnoea episodes have been noted. Closed questioning regarding night sweats, palpitations, restless sleep, acid reflux, decreased libido, impaired concentration/memory, morning headaches, how refreshed the patient feels in the morning and daytime somnolence may be required. In regard of the latter symptoms, all patients should complete the Epworth Sleepiness Scale (Table 1). Higher scores, particularly above 10, have been correlated with an increased likelihood of an OSA diagnosis.[36]

Table 1: Epworth Sleepiness Scale

How likely are you to doze off or fall asleep in the following situations, in contrast to just feeling tired? Please tick one box on each line using the following scale:

0=Would never doze

1=Slight chance of dozing

2=Moderate chance of dozing

3=High chance of dozing

Situation	0	1	2	3
Sitting and Reading				
Watching television				
Sitting inactive in public place(e.g. theatre or meeting)				
As a passenger in a car for an hour without break				
Lying down in the afternoon when circumstances permit				
Sitting and talking to someone				
Sitting quietly after lunch without alcohol				
In a car, while stopped for a few minutes in the traffic				

A full social and past medical history is necessary to ascertain the impact of smoking, alcohol and medications (e.g. sedatives) alongside an assessment of co-morbidities, not only for fitness for surgery but also to rule out contributing conditions such as hypothyroidism or acromegaly. In addition, rhinological pathology (e.g. allergic rhinitis, chronic rhinosinusitis with polyposis, septal deviation, alar collapse) should be screened for as these can also contribute to SRDB and form a limiting factor for nasal CPAP compliance.[37]

Clinical examination includes a full head and neck examination to assess for nasal pathology, tonsillar hypertrophy, soft palate and uvula dimensions, redundant pharyngeal mucosa and tongue position. Mallampati and Friedman scores can help to grade tongue position and recent literature suggests a correlation with the severity of OSA in addition to which surgical sites may be targeted for therapy (Figure 2); patients with Friedman tongue position (FTP) 1 are more likely to benefit from palatal surgery as compared to those with FTP 3/4.[38-41]

Body mass index and neck collar size should also be documented. During this general inspection, retrognathia, dental malocclusion and any obvious craniofacial abnormalities should be considered. All patients should undergo flexible nasopharyngolaryngoscopy in outpatients to dynamically assess the upper airway including the tongue base and larynx. At this juncture, simulated snoring or Muller's manoeuvre can be applied, although their value is unclear, in part due to their subjectivity.[42-44]

Figure 2: Friedman Tongue Positions.

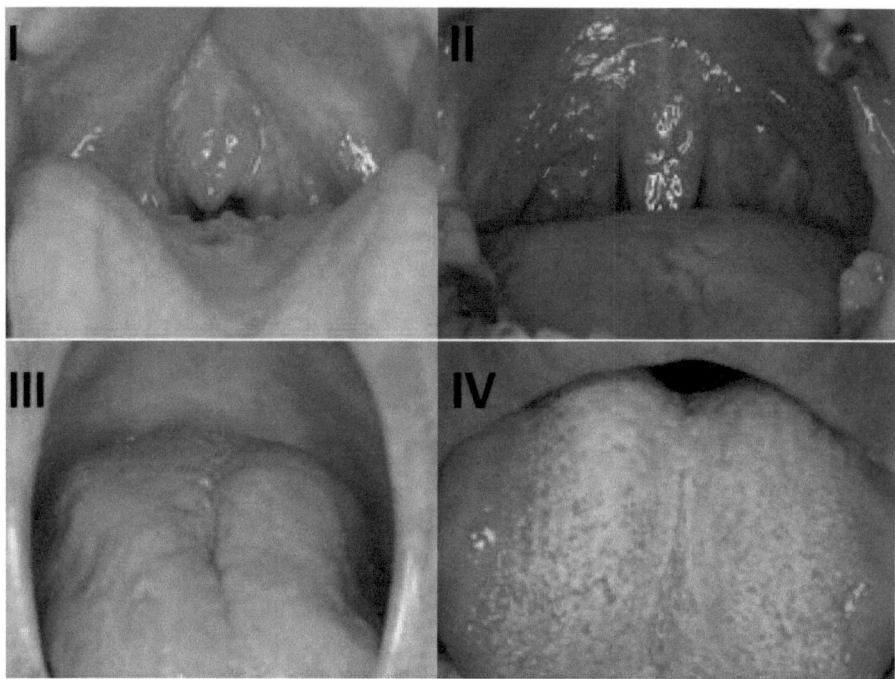

With kind permission from Springer Science and Business Media: [19]Virk JS, Nouraei R, Kotecha B. Multilevel radiofrequency ablation to the soft palate and tongue base: tips and pitfalls. Eur Arch Otorhinolaryngol 2014; 271:1809-1813.

Further investigations are then ordered dependent upon the history and examination. The gold standard investigation to diagnose OSA is a hospital-based polysomnography, although in many centres in Europe, ambulatory sleep studies are performed due to financial constraints, availability and patient preference. Objective values often analysed from these studies include apnoea/hypopnoea index (AHI), mean oxygenation and oxygen desaturation index. An apnoea has been defined as a cessation of airflow for at least ten seconds whilst a reduction in tidal volume or vital capacity by at least 30 % is a hypopnoeic episode.[1] Moreover, AHI serves as a marker of severity with mild (5-15), moderate (16-30) and severe OSA (more than 30) delineated by the index score.[1] These markers should of course be interpreted in light of the patient's age, symptoms and co-morbidities.[11,12]

Further investigations have been proposed ranging from imaging, acoustic analysis, pressure transducers and sleep nasendoscopy but all have limitations and thus have not been universally accepted.[45]

Although some controversy persists, drug-induced sedation endoscopy (DISE) or sleep nasendoscopy is now widely advocated.[46,47] The main criticism remains that drug-induced sleep differs from natural physiological sleep alongside the inherent subjectivity in assessment and lack of standardised grading systems. This is countered by the suggestion that these drugs would affect different segments equally and thus still allow evaluation of obstruction at each anatomical level. Alongside this, recent studies have confirmed superiority to awake assessment by flexible nasopharyngolaryngoscopy in outpatients and correlation with AHI, mean oxygen desaturation alongside surgical outcomes with good inter-rater reliability.[45,48-51] Moreover the recent European position paper has attempted to standardise nomenclature and data capture from these procedures.[47] As a corollary to this standardisation, the advent of a neurophysiological (bispectral index) monitoring device may indicate at which juncture DISE should be performed, potentially allowing for the development of clearer protocols and aid anaesthetists in providing appropriate sedation.[12,48]

Surgical technique

A number of radiofrequency devices are available and can be monopolar or bipolar. Modes of action, as outlined above, can be temperature or pressure-modulated, with or without feedback control such as Somnus® (Gyrus, Memphis, TN, USA), Sutter® (Fribourg, Germany), Coblator® (Arthrocare Corp, Sunnyvale, CA, USA) and Ellman® (Oceanside, NY, USA). Some act in dry whilst others in wet mediums.[19,26] Recent literature indicates that, despite differing technical characteristics, all devices have comparable efficacy with a good safety profile.[52-55] Commercially available radiofrequency generators all have slightly different characteristics in terms of wavelength, RF parameters, presence or absence of acoustic feedback, monopolar or bipolar electrode and the length of the active electrode.[54] Each therefore have their own advantages and limitations. The current Somnus® generator has an automated energy delivery system that maintains tissue temperature at a level selected by the physician, providing continuous feedback and increased control, with a clear graphical display.[56] The Sutter® Radiofrequency generator is available in monopolar or bipolar mode and has an automatic safety feature that adjusts power volume depending on tissue condition.[57] It of course therefore allows both electrosection and coagulation modes. Bipolar systems use less power, allow more precise applications and therefore create less collateral thermal damage. In addition, monopolar requires grounding pads on the patient, and may produce an unpredictable electric field in the patient's body with an associated possibility of heating metallic materials such as surgical clips or pacemakers.[58] Coblation has also demonstrated similar efficacies as other generators, with a suggestion of a potential reduced pain side effect profile in addition to the advantage of a multi-functional wand applicator that integrates saline, suction and power controls.[55,59]

We recommend the use of bipolar radiofrequency with impedance control, such as the Celon® system (Olympus, KeyMed Medical Industries and Equipment Ltd., UK), as this allows a precise defined treatment area. In addition this system generates an acoustic auto-cut off as a safety mechanism. Furthermore, the principle advantage is the use of disposable probes for both cutting and coagulation modes, without changing devices.[19]

As with any surgery, the outcome is operator dependent and as such, adequate training is required to reduce the risk of complications and optimally conduct the technique. We recommend general anaesthetic procedures due, in part, to patient preference in the UK but also to avoid a potentially moving target, as one of the important steps of the procedure is to fully insert the probe into the interstitial layer, to avoid superficial burns and hence the risk of fistulation and ulceration. In addition, from the surgeon's perspective, there is improved exposure and access with general anaesthesia (Table 2 and Figure 3).[19] This is further augmented with nasotracheal intubation for soft palate and tongue base procedures. Patients are given intravenous dexamethasone at induction.

Table 2: Tips and pitfalls.

Region	Tips	Pitfalls
Soft palate	Post-nasal packing Local anaesthetic

2nd stage – medial to lateral (for additional separate lesions)

Uvula – infiltrate with LA and bevel application

Celon® – disposable; auto cut off; cutting and coagulation modes | Blanching/superficial application – risk of ulceration/fistulation

2nd stage application – fibrosis/resistance

Uvula – more than 50% and not bevelled – can lead to nasal regurgitation or incompetence |
| Base of tongue | Nasotracheal intubation/Head up table position/Boyle-Davis Gag in situ with tongue pulled forward with Denis Browne Forceps

Simultaneous digital pressure on thyroid/cricoid (to express epiglottis into view) and mylohyoid (to visualize tongue base) | Poor view and resultant inaccurate probe insertion increasing risk of complications and poor outcomes

Local anaesthetic procedures – patient comfort, access, arrest of bleeding, accurate siting and applications with probe |

With kind permission from Springer Science and Business Media: [19]Virk JS, Nouraei R, Kotecha B. Multilevel radiofrequency ablation to the soft palate and tongue base: tips and pitfalls. Eur Arch Otorhinolaryngol 2014; 271:1809-1813.

The soft palate and oral cavity are prepared with aqueous chlorhexidine and the soft palate mucosa is infiltrated with local anaesthetic with adrenaline (2ml of 2 % Lidocaine with 1:80000 adrenaline). This serves as a haemostatic agent and increases interstitial volume, thereby facilitating access for the probe (but as the histopathological studies demonstrated, does not lead to a change in lesion size by the putative dissipation of thermal energy).[19,26,60]

Excision of redundant palatopharyngeus posterior pillar mucosa is performed with the Celon® ProCut needle at a power setting of 25 W. The same procedure is undertaken to remove excess uvula tissue, typically 50 % and bevelled, to facilitate closure of the mucosa and maintain the nasopharyngeal inlet, preventing nasal regurgitation or incompetence. Further haemostasis is not usually required but bipolar electrocautery can be used.[19,26]

Radiofrequency of the soft palate is performed by introduction of an electrode delivery device or radiofrequency probe set at 10 W and carefully directed to the palate, interstitially only. To aid in this, prior to application of local anaesthetic, tonsil swabs are inserted to serve as post-nasal space packing; this safety measure raises the soft palate thus preventing injury to the posterior pharyngeal wall and pre-vertebral fascia. Ten applications are usually undertaken with four in the median portion extending from the posterior nasal spine to the uvula base and six directed lateral to medial, ensuring an absence of blanching which is indicative of a superficial application and a resultant risk of ulceration and fistula formation (Figure 3D).[19,26]

Figure 3: Surgical procedure **A**. Standard patient position with short Boyle-Davis gag in situ, tongue protrusion and nasotracheal intubation. **B**. Optimal visualization of epiglottis and access to tongue base with additional digital pressure over mylohyoid. **C**. Radiofrequency application sites to tongue base with Celon® system. **D**. Radiofrequency application sites (*marked*) to soft palate in first stage procedure. Note use of local anaesthetic and post-nasal packing.

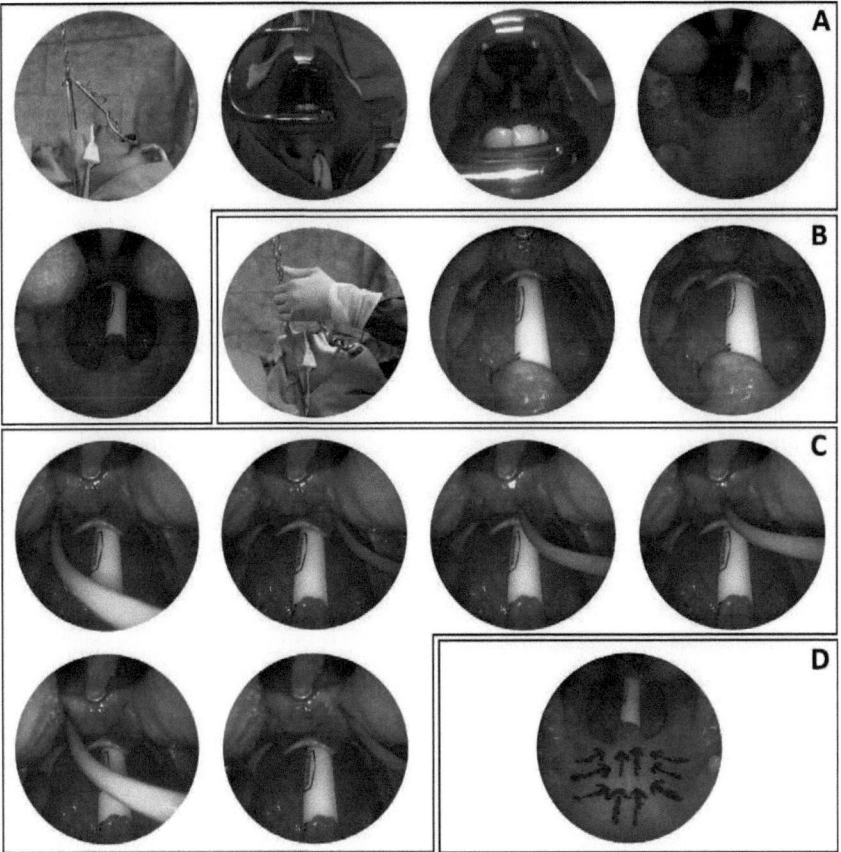

Radiofrequency to the tongue base may require additional gentle pressure over the mylohyoid to optimise the view. The same probe is used with a lower power of 6 W due to the markedly larger bulk of the tongue as compared to the soft palate. This allows for a longer application and thus a bigger lesion. Six treatments are directed perpendicular to the surface of the tongue away from the lateral border to avoid the neurovascular bundles and posterior to the circumvallate papillae (Figure 3C). The inter-lesional distance should be a minimum of 8 mm to avoid submucosal coalescence of lesions.[19,26]

The number of applications can vary and is determined by the length and breadth of the soft palate and exposure of the region posterior to the circumvallate papillae at the tongue base.

About two thirds of patients require a second stage procedure but this can be conducted as a day case or in the outpatient setting.[61-65] In second stage applications to the soft palate, the probe is directed medial to lateral to avoid overtreatment to a single area; this may lead to an additive effect of treatments in different palatal areas along with avoiding fibrosed tissue, which can be more resistant, difficult to access and hence susceptible to superficial applications and its associated complications.[19] This change in technique is not required at the base of tongue due to its larger muscle bulk.

Radiofrequency to the inferior turbinates can be necessary and this can be performed with the same interstitial probe at an appropriate power setting (15 W).[66] Previously the senior author had used a power setting of 12 W which resulted in an increase in secondary haemorrhage as lesions were fairly sizeable and so a more conservative power setting is now utilised. Care should be taken when applying the probe along the turbinate to ensure that it is not adherent to the bone of the turbinate as this could result in necrosis and haemorrhage. This highlights the multilevel nature of SRDB, although most commonly this surgery is performed to facilitate the use of nasal CPAP rather than to solely resolve the SRDB. A number of radiofrequency devices have been used with similar success rates at long term follow up for turbinate reductions, including monopolar and bipolar.[52,53] If the inferior turbinate surgery is conducted in conjunction with radiofrequency treatments to the soft palate and tongue, then the nasotracheal intubation will require changing to a laryngeal mask to allow access to the nasal cavity. This part of the multilevel surgery is therefore typically performed following applications to the tongue base and palate.

Long term outcomes

There is increasing evidence of the short to medium term efficacy of RFA for SRDB, particularly OSA and simple snoring. A recent meta-analysis verified the safety and minimal morbidity associated with radiofrequency treatments but also indicated that RFA for SRDB resulted in a significant improvement in follow up times of at least one year.[67] Farrar et al had previously documented the effectiveness of RFA in follow up times of less than one year.[68] Both reviews were limited by the quality of studies available for inclusion. A higher level of evidence is required, with robust data collection parameters and long term follow up.

Recent level 1b evidence demonstrated that RFA of the soft palate had no effect on snoring or AHI at one year follow up, in contrast to the findings of significant benefit of RFA to the soft palate in similar study of efficacy (in a placebo-controlled trial of RFA) by Stuck et al in 2005.[69,70] De Kermandec et al also found that, at six year follow up, most patients had relapse of snoring symptoms.[71] Controversy therefore persists and many other studies have refuted this, including at long term follow up of up to five years.[65,72,73] Baba et al have produced the most recent systematic review indicating the benefit of RFA at long term.[74]

Complications

Radiofrequency ablation treatments for patients with SRDB has a better side effect profile with less postoperative pain, as compared to traditional techniques such as an extensive uvulopalatoplasty.[61-65]

Specific complications of RFA include bleeding, infection, ulceration, palatal fistulation (Figure 4), tongue weakness, taste disturbance and globus sensation. Long term complications are unusual but globus sensation may persist in up to 10 % of patients.[19] In a large series, Stuck reported a complication rate of less than 1 %.[62] Recent NICE guidance confirms this safety profile.[75]

Figure 4: ulceration (black arrow) and fistulation (white arrow); note slough tissue following bilateral tonsillectomy.

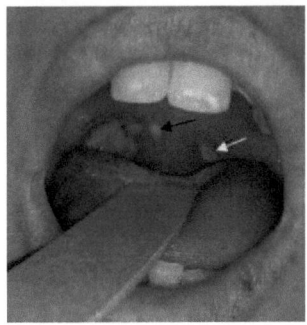

With kind permission from Springer Science and Business Media: [26]Virk JS, Kumar G, Al-Okati D, Kotecha B. Radiofrequency ablation in snoring surgery: local tissue effects and safety measures. Eur Arch Otorhinolaryngol 2014; 271:3313-3318.

The principle risk with RF to the inferior turbinates, as with most turbinoplasty procedures, is secondary haemorrhage. In an attempt to reduce this risk, a power setting in the order of 15 W in the Celon® system is recommended to potentially generate smaller lesions with less bone necrosis and tissue reaction, which can then lead to infection and secondary bleeding.

Complications that have been reported following RFA to the tongue base include ulceration, dysphagia and even more rarely, abscess or haematoma formation, which could lead to airway compromise. A unique complication that was recently recorded following tongue base RFA was thyroglossal cyst infection, and caution should be exercised when operating on patients with known remnant cysts. Indeed, as compared to the soft palate and inferior turbinate RFA procedures, the tongue base procedures do carry a higher rate of moderate and severe complications.[76,77] We recommend a multi-step consent process and provision of appropriate patient information leaflets alongside an index of suspicion, particularly in cases of tongue base RFA.

Recommendations

Radiofrequency thermal ablation surgery has been one of the most promising avenues for research for the treatment of SRDBs in the last twenty years. Its efficacy has been demonstrated over the short to medium term and the side effect profile is minimal. Current NICE guidance corroborates this safety profile.[75] It can be carried out under local or general anaesthetic.

This extensive review has highlighted specific technical considerations which will reduce complications, the importance of patient selection, and an understanding of its histopathological and collateral effects.

We therefore recommend the use of radiofrequency as a first line treatment in patients with palatal and tongue base multilevel obstruction, without epiglottic retraction (trapdoor phenomenon). All patients should be discharged with regular analgesia, a short course of steroids and mouthwash. We recommend secondary applications in patients in 2-3 months if there has been no significant improvement. Thereafter, repeat drug-induced sedation endoscopy is advised to further assess the altered dynamics of the upper airway to further select appropriate management steps.

RFA is most suited for patients with snoring or mild OSA. The gold standard of therapy for moderate to severe OSA remains CPAP.[75] However, many patients fail to tolerate CPAP and in this scenario, RFA can be used to treat the upper airway obstruction in order to increase upper airway dimensions and hence facilitate the use of CPAP, by, for example, reducing pressure requirements.

Further work

The main limitation of a number of these studies is the lack of standardisation in nomenclature and outcomes data. Drug-induced sedation endoscopy is useful as it allows visualisation of the upper airway obstruction in the dynamic mode but is often criticised due not only to a drug-induced sleep state but also because of the inherent subjectivity and lack of standardised grading systems. This has been somewhat addressed by a recent European congress meeting but a universally accepted scoring or classification system is still lacking.[47]

Likewise, the definitions of success and outcomes for these patients undergoing treatment are unclear. A combination of patient-centred and objective outcomes would be optimal but many continue to use reduction in AHI alone as an 'end-point.' This is highlighted in a recent Cochrane review and so further work is required to generate robust, long term data collated in a prospective manner alongside with the formulation of tangible and answerable trial hypotheses.[78,79]

For RFA, further research is required to confirm long term efficacy and also to investigate the histopathological effects on differing tissue over an extended time period, although this may be difficult to perform in vivo. Moreover, there is a lack of high level evidence within this field but also for surgery in general. Many therefore recommend higher volume clinical research with a more robust framework.[11,80]

Conclusion

Radiofrequency thermal ablation is increasingly recognised as a valid and effective treatment of patients with a range of sleep-related breathing disorders, with evidence of at least medium term benefit and less post-operative complications. This review provides an update of current evidence and techniques.

Acknowledgements

Thank you to Springer Science and Business Media for allowing reproduction of figures and tables originally published in their journals.

Conflicts of Interest

None

Financial declarations

We declare that in our radiological airway study (*Heywood RL, Khalil HM, Kothari S, Chawda S, Kotecha BT. Radiological airway changes following bipolar radiofrequency volumetric tissue reduction. J Laryngol Otol 2010; 124:1078-1084*) financial support from Celon® was accepted.

In addition, Olympus® UK have contributed to our radiofrequency research fund at Royal National Throat Nose and Ear Hospital.

No financial support was received for this project.

References

1.   Sleep-related breathing disorders in adults: recommendations for syndrome definition and measurement techniques in clinical research. The Report of an American Academy of Sleep Medicine Task Force. Sleep 1999; 22:667-689.

2.   Young T, Palta M, Dempsey J, Skatrud J, Weber S, Badr S. The occurrence of sleep-disordered breathing among middle-aged adults. The New England journal of medicine 1993; 328:1230-1235.

3.   Stradling JR, Crosby JH, Payne CD. Self reported snoring and daytime sleepiness in men aged 35-65 years. Thorax 1991; 46:807-810.

4.   Stradling JR, Crosby JH. Predictors and prevalence of obstructive sleep apnoea and snoring in 1001 middle aged men. Thorax 1991; 46:85-90.

5.   Hui DS, Chan JK, Ko FWet al. Prevalence of snoring and sleep-disordered breathing in a group of commercial bus drivers in Hong Kong. Internal medicine journal 2002; 32:149-157.

6.   http://www.britishsnoring.co.uk/pdf/epidem.pdf.

7.   Young T, Evans L, Finn L, Palta M. Estimation of the clinically diagnosed proportion of sleep apnea syndrome in middle-aged men and women. Sleep 1997; 20:705-706.

8.   AlGhanim N, Comondore VR, Fleetham J, Marra CA, Ayas NT. The economic impact of obstructive sleep apnea. Lung 2008; 186:7-12.

9.   Foley D, Ancoli-Israel S, Britz P, Walsh J. Sleep disturbances and chronic disease in older adults: results of the 2003 National Sleep Foundation Sleep in America Survey. Journal of psychosomatic research 2004; 56:497-502.

10. Namen AM, Dunagan DP, Fleischer Aet al. Increased physician-reported sleep apnea: the National Ambulatory Medical Care Survey. Chest 2002; 121:1741-1747.

11.   Schraufnagel D. Breathing in America: Diseases, Progress, and Hope. USA: American Thoracic Society, 2010.

12.   Virk JS, Kotecha B. Otorhinolaryngological Aspects of Sleep-Related Breathing Disorders. J Thorac Dis 2016; *in press*.

13.   George CF, Smiley A. Sleep apnea & automobile crashes. Sleep 1999; 22:790-795.

14.   He J, Kryger MH, Zorick FJ, Conway W, Roth T. Mortality and apnea index in obstructive sleep apnea. Experience in 385 male patients. Chest 1988; 94:9-14.

15.   Guilleminault C, Connolly SJ, Winkle RA. Cardiac arrhythmia and conduction disturbances during sleep in 400 patients with sleep apnea syndrome. The American journal of cardiology 1983; 52:490-494.

16.   Yaggi HK, Concato J, Kernan WN, Lichtman JH, Brass LM, Mohsenin V. Obstructive sleep apnea as a risk factor for stroke and death. The New England journal of medicine 2005; 353:2034-2041.

17.   Ip MS, Lam B, Ng MM, Lam WK, Tsang KW, Lam KS. Obstructive sleep apnea is independently associated with insulin resistance. American journal of respiratory and critical care medicine 2002; 165:670-676.

18.   Marshall NS, Wong KK, Liu PY, Cullen SR, Knuiman MW, Grunstein RR. Sleep apnea as an independent risk factor for all-cause mortality: the Busselton Health Study. Sleep 2008; 31:1079-1085.

19.   Virk JS, Nouraei R, Kotecha B. Multilevel radiofrequency ablation to the soft palate and tongue base: tips and pitfalls. European archives of oto-rhino-laryngology : official journal of the European Federation of Oto-Rhino-Laryngological Societies 2014; 271:1809-1813.

20.   Powell NB, Riley RW, Troell RJ, Li K, Blumen MB, Guilleminault C. Radiofrequency volumetric tissue reduction of the palate in subjects with sleep-disordered breathing. Chest 1998; 113:1163-1174.

21. Fischer Y, Khan M, Mann WJ. Multilevel temperature-controlled radiofrequency therapy of soft palate, base of tongue, and tonsils in adults with obstructive sleep apnea. The Laryngoscope 2003; 113:1786-1791.

22. Sandhu GS, Vatts A, Whinney D, Kotecha B, Croft CB. Somnoplasty for simple snoring--a pilot study. Clinical otolaryngology and allied sciences 2003; 28:425-429.

23. Tatla T, Sandhu G, Croft CB, Kotecha B. Celon radiofrequency thermo-ablative palatoplasty for snoring - a pilot study. The Journal of laryngology and otology 2003; 117:801-806.

24. Stimpson P, Kotecha B. Histopathological and ultrastructural effects of cutting radiofrequency energy on palatal soft tissues: a prospective study. European archives of oto-rhino-laryngology : official journal of the European Federation of Oto-Rhino-Laryngological Societies 2011; 268:1829-1836.

25. Organ LW. Electrophysiologic principles of radiofrequency lesion making. Applied neurophysiology 1976; 39:69-76.

26. Virk JS, Kumar G, Al-Okati D, Kotecha B. Radiofrequency ablation in snoring surgery: local tissue effects and safety measures. European archives of oto-rhino-laryngology : official journal of the European Federation of Oto-Rhino-Laryngological Societies 2014; 271:3313-3318.

27. Desinger K ST, Tschepe J. . Investigations on radiofrequency current application in bipolar technique for interstitial thermotherapy. Minimal Invasive Med 1996; 7:5.

28. Rathke H, Hamm B, Guttler Fet al. Comparison of four radiofrequency ablation systems at two target volumes in an ex vivo bovine liver model. Diagnostic and interventional radiology 2014; 20:251-258.

29. Desinger K ST, Mueller G. High frequency current application in bipolar technique for interstitial thermotherapy (HF-ITT). In: Anderson R BK, Bass LS,

ed. *SPOE Lasers in surgery: advanced characterisation, therapeutics and systems*. Germany, 1997:526-535.

30. De Salles AA, Brekhus SD, De Souza ECet al. Early postoperative appearance of radiofrequency lesions on magnetic resonance imaging. Neurosurgery 1995; 36:932-936; discussion 936-937.

31. Heywood RL, Khalil HM, Kothari S, Chawda S, Kotecha BT. Radiological airway changes following bipolar radiofrequency volumetric tissue reduction. The Journal of laryngology and otology 2010; 124:1078-1084.

32. Stuck BA, Kopke J, Maurer JTet al. Lesion formation in radiofrequency surgery of the tongue base. The Laryngoscope 2003; 113:1572-1576.

33. Powell NB, Riley RW, Troell RJ, Blumen MB, Guilleminault C. Radiofrequency volumetric reduction of the tongue. A porcine pilot study for the treatment of obstructive sleep apnea syndrome. Chest 1997; 111:1348-1355.

34. MA DA. Action physiologique des courants alternatifs. CR Soc Biol 1891; 43:3.

35. VA MJaVR. History of Ablation. In: van Sonnenberg E MWaSL, ed. *Tumour Ablation*. New York: Springer, 2005:3-16.

36. Johns MW. A new method for measuring daytime sleepiness: the Epworth sleepiness scale. Sleep 1991; 14:540-545.

37. Kotecha B. The nose, snoring and obstructive sleep apnoea. Rhinology 2011; 49:259-263.

38. Mallampati SR, Gatt SP, Gugino LDet al. A clinical sign to predict difficult tracheal intubation: a prospective study. Canadian Anaesthetists' Society journal 1985; 32:429-434.

39. Friedman M, Hamilton C, Samuelson CG, Lundgren ME, Pott T. Diagnostic value of the Friedman tongue position and Mallampati classification for obstructive sleep apnea: a meta-analysis. Otolaryngology--head and neck surgery : official journal of American Academy of Otolaryngology-Head and Neck Surgery 2013; 148:540-547.

40. Friedman M, Ibrahim H, Bass L. Clinical staging for sleep-disordered breathing. Otolaryngology--head and neck surgery : official journal of American Academy of Otolaryngology-Head and Neck Surgery 2002; 127:13-21.

41. Friedman M, Ibrahim H, Joseph NJ. Staging of obstructive sleep apnea/hypopnea syndrome: a guide to appropriate treatment. The Laryngoscope 2004; 114:454-459.

42. Herzog M, Metz T, Schmidt Aet al. The prognostic value of simulated snoring in awake patients with suspected sleep-disordered breathing: introduction of a new technique of examination. Sleep 2006; 29:1456-1462.

43. Ritter CT, Trudo FJ, Goldberg AN, Welch KC, Maislin G, Schwab RJ. Quantitative evaluation of the upper airway during nasopharyngoscopy with the Muller maneuver. The Laryngoscope 1999; 109:954-963.

44. Tuncel U, Inancli HM, Kurkcuoglu SS, Enoz M. Can the Muller maneuver detect multilevel obstruction of the upper airway in patients with obstructive sleep apnea syndrome? Kulak burun bogaz ihtisas dergisi : KBB = Journal of ear, nose, and throat 2010; 20:84-88.

45. Georgalas C, Garas G, Hadjihannas E, Oostra A. Assessment of obstruction level and selection of patients for obstructive sleep apnoea surgery: an evidence-based approach. The Journal of laryngology and otology 2010; 124:1-9.

46. Gupta S, Nicoli T, Kotecha B. Latest trends in the assessment and surgical management of snoring in England: a prospective questionnaire study. Clinical otolaryngology : official journal of ENT-UK ; official journal of Netherlands Society for Oto-Rhino-Laryngology & Cervico-Facial Surgery 2014; 39:177-182.

47. De Vito A, Carrasco Llatas M, Vanni Aet al. European position paper on drug-induced sedation endoscopy (DISE). Sleep & breathing = Schlaf & Atmung 2014; 18:453-465.

48. Abdullah VJ, Lee DL, Ha SC, van Hasselt CA. Sleep endoscopy with midazolam: sedation level evaluation with bispectral analysis. Otolaryngology--head and neck surgery : official journal of American Academy of Otolaryngology-Head and Neck Surgery 2013; 148:331-337.

49. Croft CB, Pringle M. Sleep nasendoscopy: a technique of assessment in snoring and obstructive sleep apnoea. Clinical otolaryngology and allied sciences 1991; 16:504-509.

50. Georgalas C, Kotecha B. Predictive value of sleep nasendoscopy in the management of habitual snorers. The Annals of otology, rhinology, and laryngology 2004; 113:420.

51. Kotecha BT, Hannan SA, Khalil HM, Georgalas C, Bailey P. Sleep nasendoscopy: a 10-year retrospective audit study. European archives of oto-rhino-laryngology : official journal of the European Federation of Oto-Rhino-Laryngological Societies 2007; 264:1361-1367.

52. Hytonen ML, Back LJ, Malmivaara AV, Roine RP. Radiofrequency thermal ablation for patients with nasal symptoms: a systematic review of effectiveness and complications. European archives of oto-rhino-laryngology : official journal of the European Federation of Oto-Rhino-Laryngological Societies 2009; 266:1257-1266.

53. Cavaliere M, Mottola G, Iemma M. Monopolar and bipolar radiofrequency thermal ablation of inferior turbinates: 20-month follow-up. Otolaryngology--head and neck surgery : official journal of American Academy of Otolaryngology-Head and Neck Surgery 2007; 137:256-263.

54. Blumen MB, Chalumeau F, Gauthier A, Bobin S, Coste A, Chabolle F. Comparative study of four radiofrequency generators for the treatment of snoring. Otolaryngology--head and neck surgery : official journal of American Academy of Otolaryngology-Head and Neck Surgery 2008; 138:294-299.

55. Milkov M NP, Tonchev T, Kirox F, Madjova H. Usage of Coblator-2 and ENT Celon systems for soft palate reduction in habitual snoring patients. Sleep Medicine 2013; 14:1.

56. http://www.doctorgallardo.com/extra_files/somnoplasty_equipment.pdf.

57. http://www.sutter-med.de/products/radiofrequency-generators/bm-780-ii-sets-en/faq.

58. Clasen S, Schmidt D, Boss Aet al. Multipolar radiofrequency ablation with internally cooled electrodes: experimental study in ex vivo bovine liver with mathematic modeling. Radiology 2006; 238:881-890.

59. Tvinnereim M, Mitic S, Hansen RK. Plasma radiofrequency preceded by pressure recording enhances success for treating sleep-related breathing disorders. The Laryngoscope 2007; 117:731-736.

60. Virk JS, Kotecha B. Sneezing during drug-induced sedation endoscopy. Sleep Breath 2014; 18:451-452.

61. Back LJ, Hytonen ML, Roine RP, Malmivaara AO. Radiofrequency ablation treatment of soft palate for patients with snoring: a systematic review of effectiveness and adverse effects. The Laryngoscope 2009; 119:1241-1250.

62. Back LJ, Liukko T, Sinkkonen ST, Ylikoski J, Makitie AA. Complication rates of radiofrequency surgery in the upper airways: a single institution experience. Acta oto-laryngologica 2009; 129:1469-1473.

63. Badia L, Malik N, Lund VJ, Kotecha BT. The effect of laser assisted uvulopalatoplasty on the sense of smell and taste. Rhinology 2001; 39:103-106.

64. Baisch A, Maurer JT, Hormann K, Stuck BA. Combined radiofrequency assisted uvulopalatoplasty in the treatment of snoring. European archives of oto-rhino-laryngology : official journal of the European Federation of Oto-Rhino-Laryngological Societies 2009; 266:125-130.

65.   Stuck BA. Radiofrequency-assisted uvulopalatoplasty for snoring: Long-term follow-up. The Laryngoscope 2009; 119:1617-1620.

66.   Powell NB, Zonato AI, Weaver EMet al. Radiofrequency treatment of turbinate hypertrophy in subjects using continuous positive airway pressure: a randomized, double-blind, placebo-controlled clinical pilot trial. The Laryngoscope 2001; 111:1783-1790.

67.   Veer V, Yang WY, Green R, Kotecha B. Long-term safety and efficacy of radiofrequency ablation in the treatment of sleep disordered breathing: a meta-analysis. European archives of oto-rhino-laryngology : official journal of the European Federation of Oto-Rhino-Laryngological Societies 2014; 271:2863-2870.

68.   Farrar J, Ryan J, Oliver E, Gillespie MB. Radiofrequency ablation for the treatment of obstructive sleep apnea: a meta-analysis. The Laryngoscope 2008; 118:1878-1883.

69.   Holmlund T, Levring-Jaghagen E, Franklin KA, Lindkvist M, Berggren D. Effects of Radiofrequency versus sham surgery of the soft palate on daytime sleepiness. The Laryngoscope 2014; 124:2422-2426.

70.   Stuck BA, Sauter A, Hormann K, Verse T, Maurer JT. Radiofrequency surgery of the soft palate in the treatment of snoring. A placebo-controlled trial. Sleep 2005; 28:847-850.

71.   De Kermadec H, Blumen MB, Engalenc D, Vezina JP, Chabolle F. Radiofrequency of the soft palate for sleep-disordered breathing: a 6-year follow-up study. European annals of otorhinolaryngology, head and neck diseases 2014; 131:27-31.

72.   De Vito A, Frassineti S, Panatta ML, Montevecchi F, Canzi P, Vicini C. Multilevel radiofrequency ablation for snoring and OSAHS patients therapy: long-term outcomes. European archives of oto-rhino-laryngology : official journal of the

European Federation of Oto-Rhino-Laryngological Societies 2012; 269:321-330.

73. Simunjak B, Slipac J, Krmpotic P, Dubravcic-Simunjak S. Efficiency of radiofrequency assisted uvulopalatopharyngoplasty in the treatment of snoring. Acta clinica Croatica 2011; 50:357-360.

74. Baba RY, Mohan A, Metta VV, Mador MJ. Temperature controlled radiofrequency ablation at different sites for treatment of obstructive sleep apnea syndrome: a systematic review and meta-analysis. Sleep & breathing = Schlaf & Atmung 2015; 19:891-910.

75. NICE. Interventional procedure overview of radiofrequency ablation of the soft palate for snoring. NICE 2013.

76. Tornari C, Wong G, Arora A, Kotecha B. A unique complication of radiofrequency therapy to the tongue base. International journal of surgery case reports 2015; 8C:9-12.

77. Kezirian EJ, Powell NB, Riley RW, Hester JE. Incidence of complications in radiofrequency treatment of the upper airway. The Laryngoscope 2005; 115:1298-1304.

78. Field CJ, Robinson S, Mackay S, Harrison JD, Marshall NS. Clinical equipoise in sleep surgery: investigating clinical trial targets. Otolaryngology--head and neck surgery : official journal of American Academy of Otolaryngology-Head and Neck Surgery 2011; 145:347-353.

79. Sundaram S, Bridgman SA, Lim J, Lasserson TJ. Surgery for obstructive sleep apnoea. The Cochrane database of systematic reviews 2005:CD001004.

80. Franklin KA, Anttila H, Axelsson S et al. Effects and side-effects of surgery for snoring and obstructive sleep apnea--a systematic review. Sleep 2009; 32:27-36.

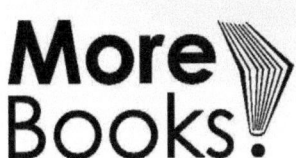
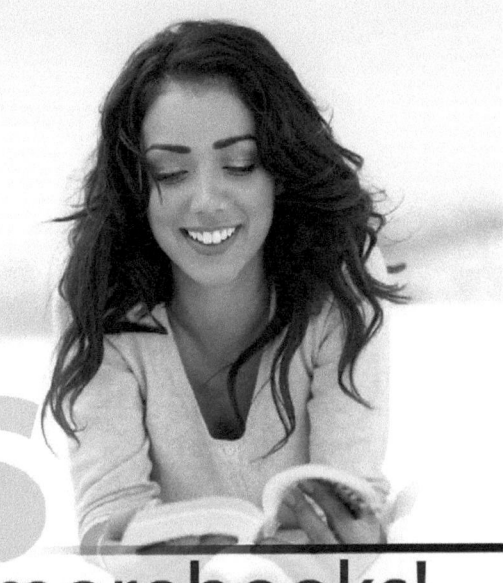 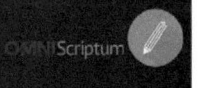

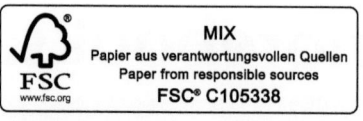
Printed by Books on Demand GmbH, Norderstedt / Germany